Breathing Exercise Buteyko Logbook

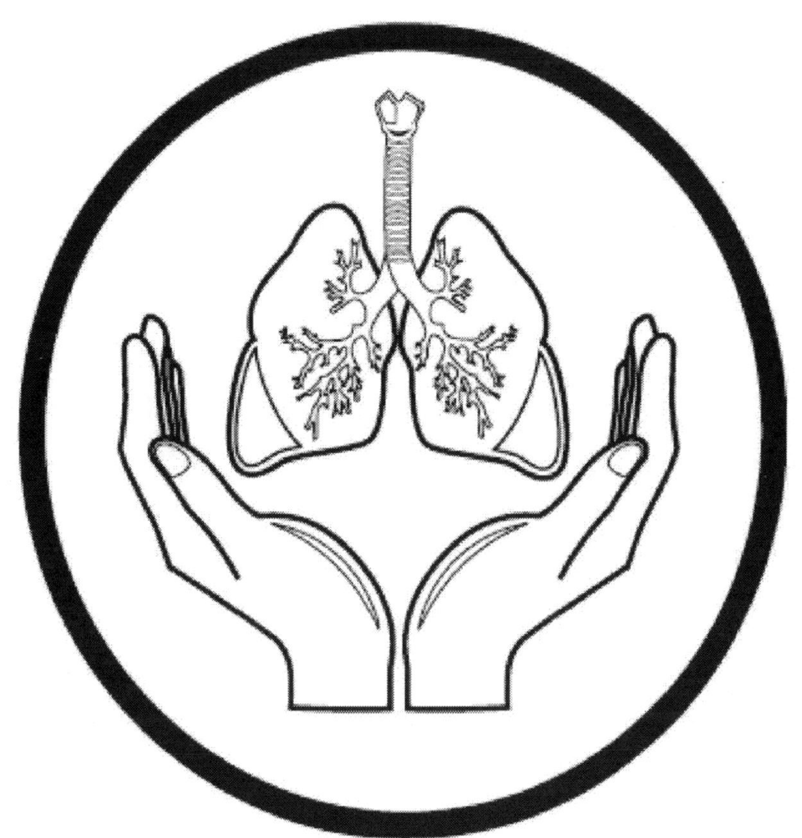

by Sasha Yakovleva

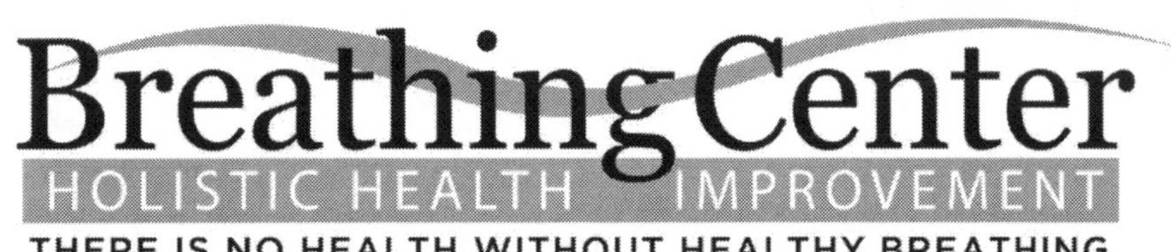

THERE IS NO HEALTH WITHOUT HEALTHY BREATHING

Breathing Center Publications
www.BreathingCenter.com—info@breathingcenter.com

ISBN: 978-151771824-4

Printed in the USA

CONTENTS

How to use this logbook:

To apply the Buteyko Breathing Normalization method correctly, a student needs to document breathing measurements. This book will help you accomplish this task. Please present this book every time you meet with your Breathing Normalization specialist. Based on the results recorded in your logbook, a practitioner will adjust your exercises to ensure optimal results.

You will need to do three formal sessions of breathing exercises every day, preferably in the morning, the middle of the day and before going to bed. Each session of breathing exercises should be about 30 minutes long (it can be shorter but not longer).

Every seated session starts with relaxation (5-10 min) and continues with breath holds (20-25 min). For relaxation, we recommend using Breathing Normalization meditations, which are available through Breathing Center's website. If it is a session in motion, relaxation could be skipped. To determine the appropriate length of breath holds, please consult with your practitioner.

To record your breathing data, you will need to measure your Control Pause (CP) or Positive Maximum Pause (PMP). Usually, students measure their CP in the beginning of their training and switch to measuring PMP when CP becomes stable on the level above 20 sec. To understand how to measure CP/PMP, please visit the Breathing Test page of Breathing Center's website (www.breathingcenter.com) or watch the 1st disc of the DVD, "*The Breathing Normalization Method*".

What measurements to record in this book?

1. **Morning CP or PMP:** Each morning, measure your CP or PMP. This is the most important data of the day, which reflects significant shifts in your habitual breathing patterns.

2. **Before CP or PMP:** Measure your CP/PMP before and after each formal session of breathing exercises. This will help to ensure that you are doing the exercises correctly. If your CP/PMP is higher after doing the exercises, then you have done them successfully. Conversely, if your CP or PMP is lower after doing the breathing exercises, then you have done them incorrectly. If this is the case, consult with your Breathing Normalization specialist to correct your technique.

3. **Breath Holds:** For each session, you will do a series of breath-holds. Make a notation of the number of breath holds and their length in the "notes" section of this logbook (where it says "1st Session," "2nd Session," and "3rd Session").

4. **Weekly Charts** are shown on double-page spreads inside this book, with the First Session on a left-hand page and the Second and Third Sessions on the adjacent right-hand page. Use the blank sections beside and beneath each chart to make **Progress Notes** about your progress and to write down any questions you have for your Breathing Normalization specialist.

How to read breathing measurements?

Please refer to the following chart created by K.P. Buteyko MD to gain a general understanding of your measurements. For precise interpretation of your breathing data, please see your Breathing Normalization specialist.

The Body Conditions and Criteria of Lung Ventilation According to Dr. Buteyko:

HEALTH STATUS	BREATHING	DEGREE OF ABNORMALITY	CO2 in ALVEOLI % (millimeters of mercury)		POSITIVE MAXIMUM PAUSE (seconds)	PULSE (beats per minute)
Super Endurance Longevity	General	VII	Special Conditions			
		VI				
		V	7.5	53.5	180	48
		IV	7.4	52.8	150	50
		III	7.3	52	120	52
		II	7.1	50.6	100	55
		I	6.8	48.5	80	57
The Norm (Optimal Health)			6.5	46.3	60	60
Disease	Excessive	I	6	42.8	50	65
		II	5.5	39.2	40	70
		III	5	35.7	30	75
		IV	4.5	32.1	20	80
		V	4	28.5	10	90
		VII	3.5	25	5	100
VII DEATH						

Please note that an in-take of steroids and some other medical drugs might affect a proper breathing measurement. Steroids always inflate CP and PMP. If you're on steroids, keep in mind that your real measurements are significantly lower compared to what your breathing indicates.

Brief interpretation of the chart:

The norm:

According to Dr. Buteyko, a totally healthy person has morning Positive Maximum Pause of 60 seconds and Control Pause of 30 seconds or higher. This means that for this person it is easy to stay without air for one minute and extremely easy to do it for a half of a minute. At this point, a person does not have any symptoms and his immune system protects him or her from seasonal respiratory problems as well as many serious health issues. Also, his energy capacity is high and his body does not require a great deal of food or sleep in order to rejuvenate. Of course, this state of 'perfect health' does not occur when your PMP reaches 60 seconds just once. A person belongs to this category only when his PMP is 60 seconds or higher all the time – day and night – for at least six months.

In today's world, it is extremely rare to meet an individual who belongs to this category. Since 'optimal health' has become such a rarity, doctors in Clinica Buteyko (Moscow) suggested lowering 'the Buteyko norm' to 40 seconds to adjust it to our current situation.

If your PMP and CP are below the norm, it means that your health is compromised to some degree.

1st Level of Hyperventilation:
If your morning PMP is stable between 40 and 60 seconds, it means that, by modern standards, you are an extremely healthy person. Most likely, you don't have any symptoms, and even if you do they don't last long. Most likely, you must be medication-free. The problem is that your immune system is still not strong enough to completely protect you from diseases. If you develop a disease, your immune system will be weakened, which will in turn lower your PMP/ CP.

2nd Level of Hyperventilation:
If your morning PMP is in the range of 25-40 seconds, you belong to a category of the semi-healthy/semi-ill. You might actually think of yourself as a healthy person and if so, this means that you have health issues you are not aware of or consider them normal. If your PMP is closer to 25 seconds, you might still have primary symptoms of various diseases.

3rd Level of Hyperventilation:
If your PMP is between 10-25 seconds, you are not healthy. You breathe in 3-6 times more air than your body needs. This creates a very negative impact on all systems of your body and offsets many functions. Most likely, your symptoms are active and your energy level is low. It is also possible that you often experience a lack of mental clarity or have difficulties concentrating. You are influenced by weather changes.

4th Level of Hyperventilation:
Dr. Buteyko stated: if PMP is below 10 sec, a person is severely ill – whether he/she is a child or adult, whether he has symptoms or not, whether he is aware of it or not. A person from this category is emotionally vulnerable; that person's memory is not that good, neither is their ability to focus. Often there is an issue with self-esteem. This person might experience chronic fatigue or depression, or might often have small injuries. There might be severe symptoms, and the person might be on strong medication. This person critically needs to improve breathing. If they don't, the situation might get out of control to a point when it becomes difficult to correct it.

5th Level of Hyperventilation: If a person's PMP is below 5 sec, he or she is critically ill – whether he has symptoms or not. This situation needs the immediate attention of a Breathing Normalization Specialist and a lot of one-on-one work.

The last line of the chart:
When a person passes away, his/ her CP and PMP becomes zero.

You probably noticed that there is also an **upper part to Buteyko's chart**. What happens when PMP goes above the norm? Is it even possible? Yes. Many of Dr. Buteyko's students had PMP of 120 and even 180 seconds, and you can train yourself to go that far. From Buteyko's medical perspective, this state is abnormal, but in a positive way. When PMP goes beyond 60 seconds, the person often starts developing extraordinary abilities; for example, their intuition becomes stronger, their inner monolog quiets down, confidence strengthens and the decision-making process becomes easier. High PMP also reassures a disease-free state, and a long and active life.

Please keep in mind that the Breathing Normalization method is not a pill and it will not change your health instantaneously. It takes at least six months for immune, nervous and other bodily systems to rehabilitate. The Breathing Normalization training facilitates this process, but there is no way to jump from being an invalid to being a superman. Recovery is a gradual process; even though the Buteyko® method is the most effective and fastest compared to many healing techniques, it still requires time. Please be patient and diligent in your exercises! If your health is seriously impaired, most likely your PMP won't reach 60 seconds soon. It does not matter; what is important is that your Positive Maximum Pause and Control Pause will be rising, and you will be following the path to perfect health.

Example of Recordings

Example of Recordings:

Date	Day of Week	Morning CP/PMP	Before CP/PMP	1st Session	After CP/PMP
2/26	*Tue*	*CP: 3 sec*	*CP: 5 sec*	*30 min: Relax+BHs fixed BHs: 4 sec*	*CP: 7 sec*
2/27	*Wed*	*CP: 5 sec*	*CP: 6 sec*	*30 min: Relax+BHs Flexible BHs: 3-8 sec*	*CP: 9 sec*

Before CP/PMP	2nd Session	After CP/PMP
CP: *4 sec*	*20 min: Relax+BHs Fixed* *BHs: 3 sec*	*CP:* *4 sec*
CP: *7 sec*	*10 min: just BHs* *Flexible: 6-9 sec*	*CP:* *6 sec*

Before CP/PMP	3rd Session	After CP/PMP
CP: *5 sec*	*30 min: Relax+BHs* *Flexible BHs: 3-6 sec*	*CP:* *8 sec*
CP: *5 sec*	*30 min: Relax+BHs* *Fixed BHs: 5 sec*	*CP:* *7 sec*

NOTES:

Date	Day of week	Morning CP/PMP	Before CP/ PMP	1st Session	After CP/ PMP

Before CP/ PMP	2nd Session	After CP/ PMP	Before CP/ PMP	3rd Session	After CP/ PMP

NOTES:

NOTES:

Date	Day of week	Morning CP/PMP	Before CP/ PMP	1st Session	After CP/ PMP

Before CP/ PMP	2nd Session	After CP/ PMP	Before CP/ PMP	3rd Session	After CP/ PMP

NOTES:

NOTES:

Date	Day of week	Morning CP/PMP	Before CP/ PMP	1st Session	After CP/ PMP

Before CP/ PMP	2nd Session	After CP/ PMP	Before CP/ PMP	3rd Session	After CP/ PMP

NOTES:

NOTES:

Date	Day of week	Morning CP/PMP	Before CP/ PMP	1st Session	After CP/ PMP

Before CP/ PMP	2nd Session	After CP/ PMP	Before CP/ PMP	3rd Session	After CP/ PMP

NOTES:

NOTES:

Date	Day of week	Morning CP/PMP	Before CP/ PMP	1st Session	After CP/ PMP

Before CP/ PMP	2nd Session	After CP/ PMP	Before CP/ PMP	3rd Session	After CP/ PMP

NOTES:

NOTES:

Date	Day of week	Morning CP/PMP	Before CP/ PMP	1st Session	After CP/ PMP

Before CP/ PMP	2nd Session	After CP/ PMP	Before CP/ PMP	3rd Session	After CP/ PMP

NOTES:

NOTES:

Date	Day of week	Morning CP/PMP	Before CP/ PMP	1st Session	After CP/ PMP

Before CP/ PMP	2nd Session	After CP/ PMP	Before CP/ PMP	3rd Session	After CP/ PMP

NOTES:

NOTES:

Date	Day of week	Morning CP/PMP	Before CP/ PMP	1st Session	After CP/ PMP

Before CP/ PMP	2nd Session	After CP/ PMP	Before CP/ PMP	3rd Session	After CP/ PMP

NOTES:

NOTES:

Date	Day of week	Morning CP/PMP	Before CP/ PMP	1st Session	After CP/ PMP

Before CP/ PMP	2nd Session	After CP/ PMP	Before CP/ PMP	3rd Session	After CP/ PMP

NOTES:

NOTES:

Date	Day of week	Morning CP/PMP	Before CP/ PMP	1st Session	After CP/ PMP

Before CP/ PMP	2nd Session	After CP/ PMP	Before CP/ PMP	3rd Session	After CP/ PMP

NOTES:

NOTES:

Date	Day of week	Morning CP/PMP	Before CP/ PMP	1st Session	After CP/ PMP

Before CP/ PMP	2nd Session	After CP/ PMP	Before CP/ PMP	3rd Session	After CP/ PMP

NOTES:

NOTES:

Date	Day of week	Morning CP/PMP	Before CP/ PMP	1st Session	After CP/ PMP

Before CP/ PMP	2nd Session	After CP/ PMP	Before CP/ PMP	3rd Session	After CP/ PMP

NOTES:

NOTES:

Date	Day of week	Morning CP/PMP	Before CP/ PMP	1st Session	After CP/ PMP

Before CP/ PMP	2nd Session	After CP/ PMP	Before CP/ PMP	3rd Session	After CP/ PMP

NOTES:

NOTES:

Date	Day of week	Morning CP/PMP	Before CP/ PMP	1st Session	After CP/ PMP

Before CP/ PMP	2nd Session	After CP/ PMP	Before CP/ PMP	3rd Session	After CP/ PMP

NOTES:

NOTES:

Date	Day of week	Morning CP/PMP	Before CP/ PMP	1st Session	After CP/ PMP

Before CP/ PMP	2nd Session	After CP/ PMP	Before CP/ PMP	3rd Session	After CP/ PMP

NOTES:

NOTES:

Date	Day of week	Morning CP/PMP	Before CP/ PMP	1st Session	After CP/ PMP

Before CP/ PMP	2nd Session	After CP/ PMP	Before CP/ PMP	3rd Session	After CP/ PMP

NOTES:

NOTES:

Date	Day of week	Morning CP/PMP	Before CP/ PMP	1st Session	After CP/ PMP

Before CP/ PMP	2nd Session	After CP/ PMP	Before CP/ PMP	3rd Session	After CP/ PMP

NOTES:

NOTES:

Date	Day of week	Morning CP/PMP	Before CP/ PMP	1st Session	After CP/ PMP

Before CP/ PMP	2nd Session	After CP/ PMP	Before CP/ PMP	3rd Session	After CP/ PMP

NOTES:

NOTES:

Date	Day of week	Morning CP/PMP	Before CP/ PMP	1st Session	After CP/ PMP

Before CP/ PMP	2nd Session	After CP/ PMP	Before CP/ PMP	3rd Session	After CP/ PMP

NOTES:

NOTES:

Date	Day of week	Morning CP/PMP	Before CP/ PMP	1st Session	After CP/ PMP

Before CP/ PMP	2nd Session	After CP/ PMP	Before CP/ PMP	3rd Session	After CP/ PMP

NOTES:

NOTES:

Date	Day of week	Morning CP/PMP	Before CP/ PMP	1st Session	After CP/ PMP

Before CP/ PMP	2nd Session	After CP/ PMP	Before CP/ PMP	3rd Session	After CP/ PMP

NOTES:

NOTES:

Date	Day of week	Morning CP/PMP	Before CP/ PMP	1st Session	After CP/ PMP

Before CP/ PMP	2nd Session	After CP/ PMP	Before CP/ PMP	3rd Session	After CP/ PMP

NOTES:

Useful Reminders:

Never Breathe Through Your Mouth!

Avoid Over-Breathing!

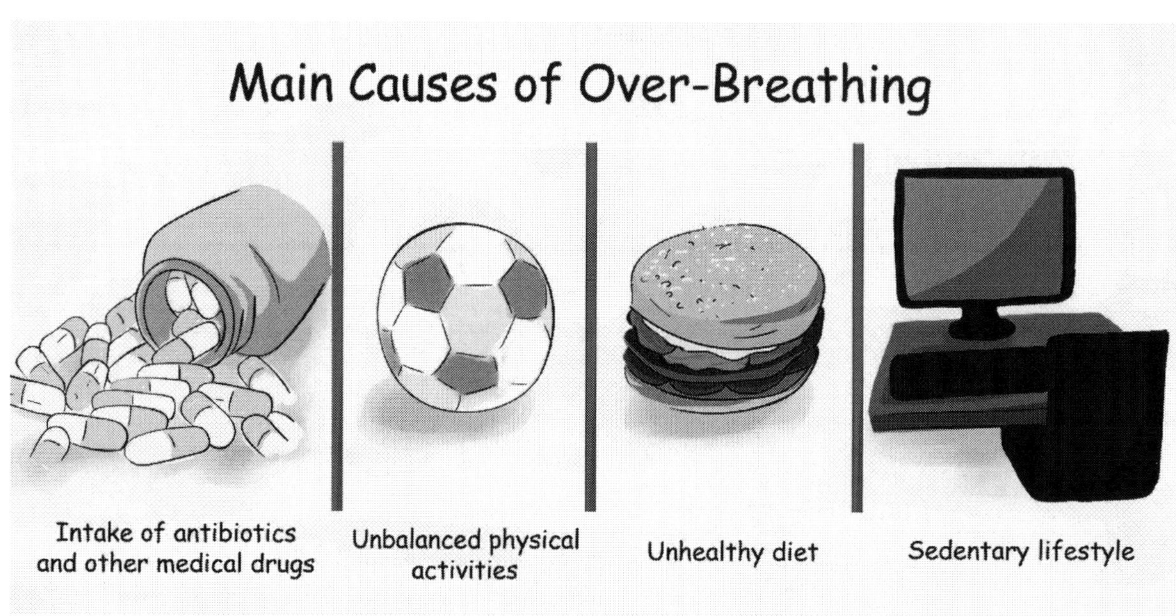

Always breathe through your nose while sleeping:

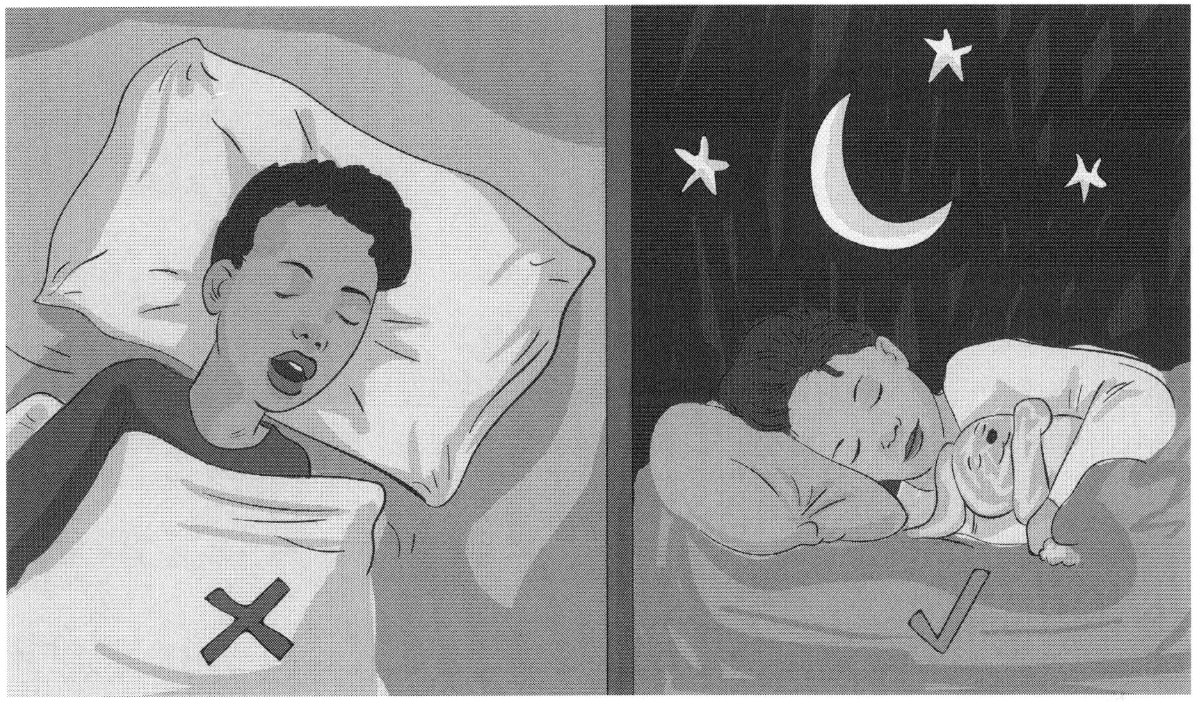

Always breathe through your nose while exercising:

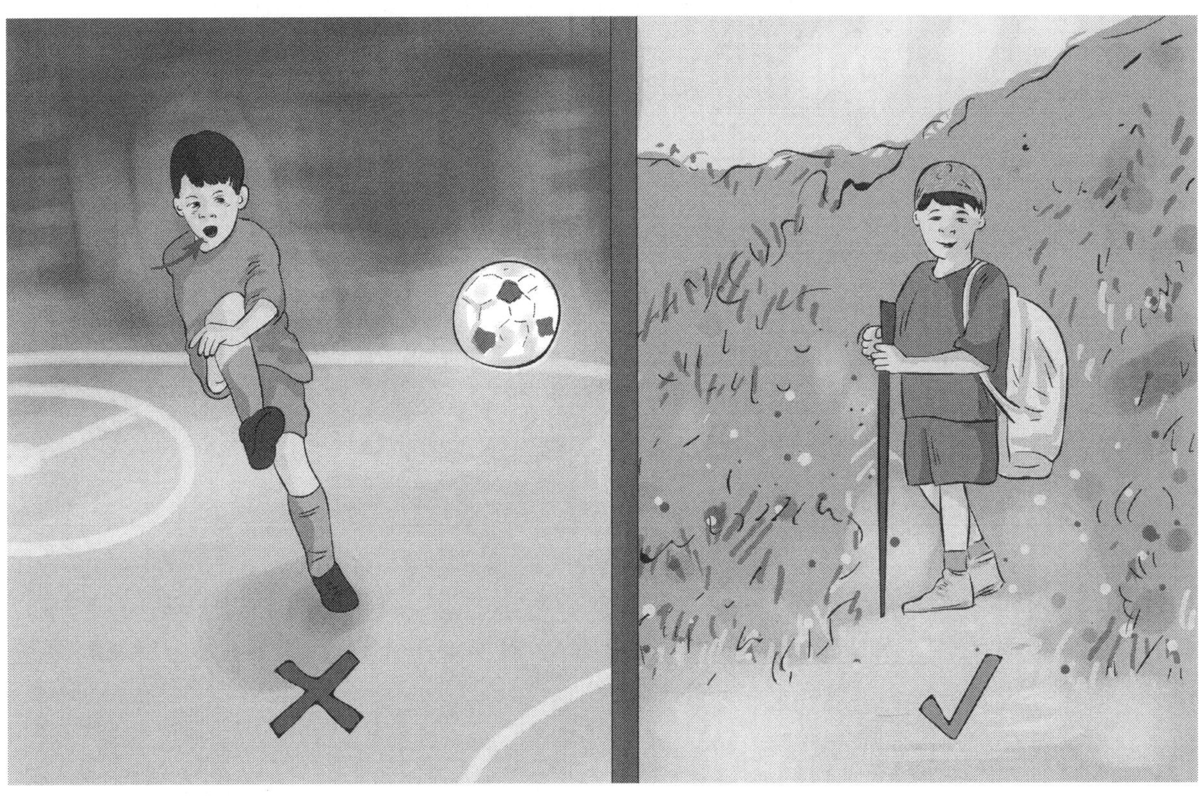

Chose a diet supportive of healthy breathing:

COLA
7up
WATER

Remember: healthy breathing is invisible

Please remember: healthy breathing is invisible.
Mom, your chest is moving!
Squirrel, your shoulders are moving!
Dad, your stomach is moving!

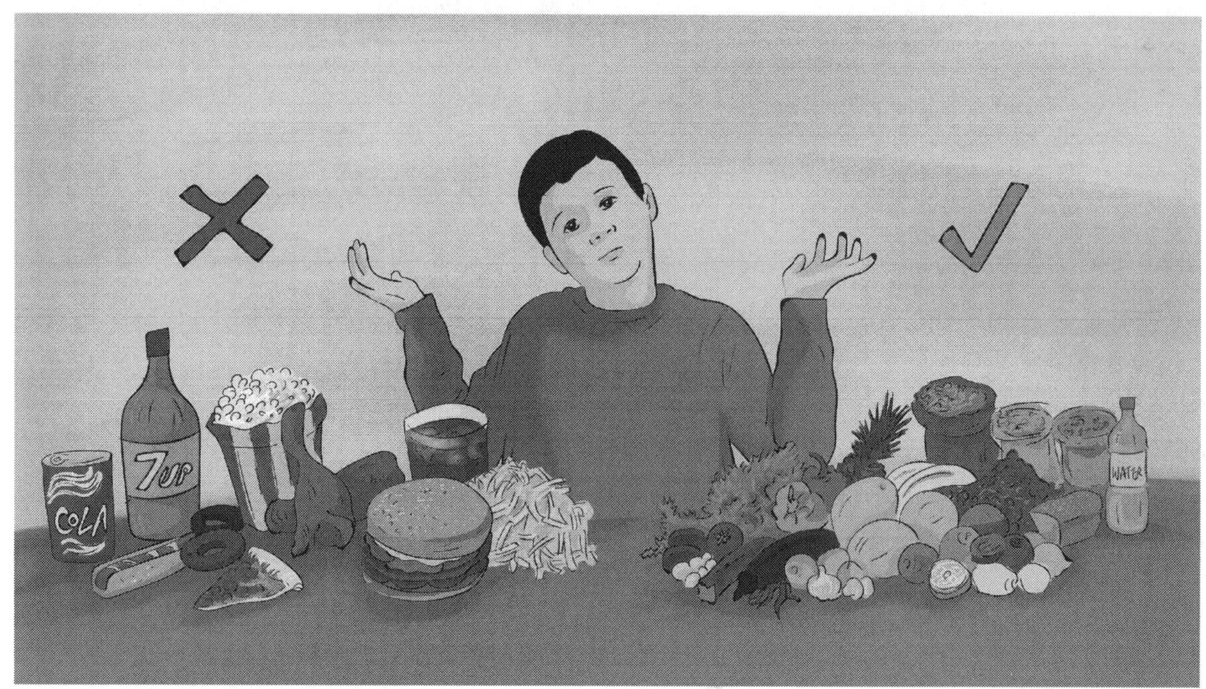

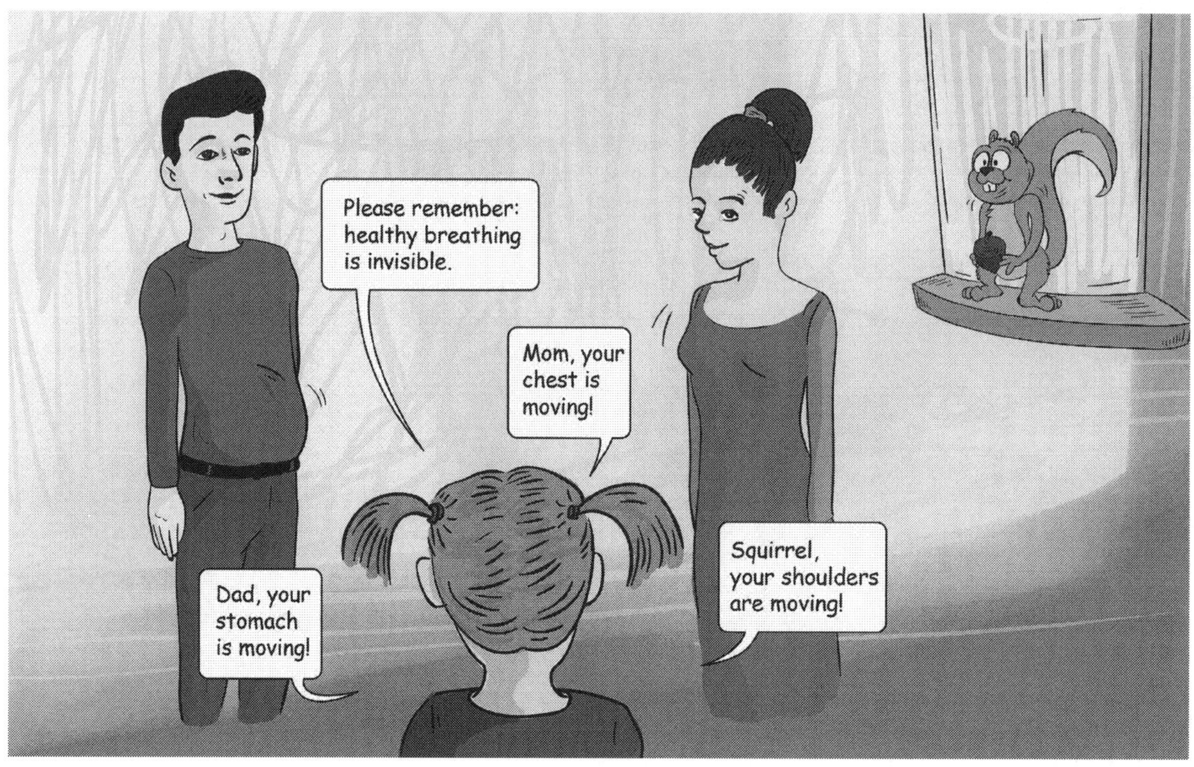

Always do your breathing exercises!

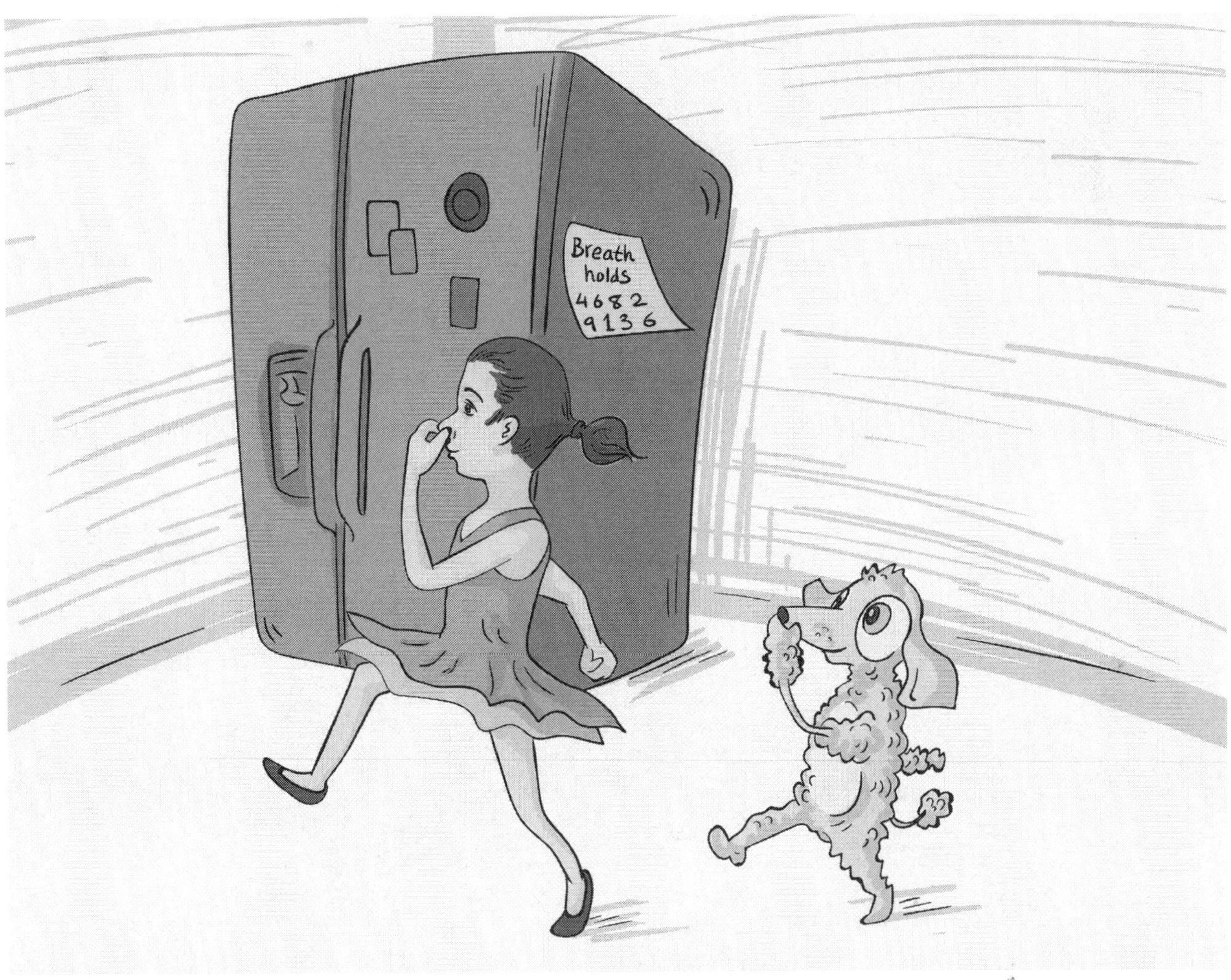

Made in United States
Orlando, FL
28 May 2024